GAIN

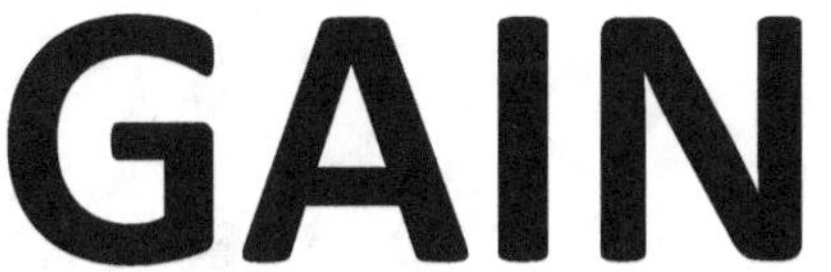

WEIGHT

CONFIDENCE

Gaining Body Weight, Body Confidence the Right way

Kevin U. Warsh Ph.D.

Table of Contents

PREFACE

Weight gain is a topic that is often discussed in the context of weight loss, but it is equally important for individuals who are underweight or trying to gain muscle mass. While being underweight can be due to genetic factors, it can also be a result of poor nutrition, lack of exercise, and other lifestyle choices. In addition to affecting one's physical appearance, being underweight can have negative impacts on overall health, such as a weakened immune system, decreased bone density, and fertility issues.

In this guide, we will explore the various factors that contribute to weight gain, including the importance of proper hydration and meal timing, exercise, and lifestyle changes. We will also address some of the common challenges that individuals face when trying to gain weight, such as finding the right balance between consuming enough calories and maintaining a healthy diet.

By understanding the underlying causes of weight gain and adopting healthy habits, individuals can achieve their weight goals and improve their overall health and wellbeing. Whether you are underweight or looking to build muscle mass, this guide will provide you with the information and tools you need to succeed on your weight gain journey.

INTRODUCTION

Weight gain is a complex topic that affects a significant portion of the population, with people striving to achieve their desired body weight for a variety of reasons. While obesity is a significant public health issue, some individuals struggle with being underweight, which can lead to various health concerns. In this introduction, we will explore the reasons behind underweight, the importance of hydration and proper meal planning, and the changes and challenges that people trying to gain weight face.

Firstly, understanding the reasons behind underweight is essential. There are several factors that contribute to being underweight, including genetics, metabolism, and lifestyle choices. Some people have a naturally thin body type, which may make it challenging to gain weight. Others may have a high metabolism that makes it difficult to put on weight. Lifestyle factors such as stress, inadequate sleep, and physical activity can also affect weight gain. Certain medical conditions, such as thyroid problems, gastrointestinal disorders, and eating disorders, can also lead to being underweight.

While proper hydration and meal planning are essential for weight gain, individuals face unique changes and challenges when trying to gain weight. For some, gaining weight can be a difficult and frustrating process. It can be challenging to consume enough calories and nutrients to promote weight gain, particularly for those who have a small appetite or a high metabolism. Additionally, gaining weight can be expensive, as it may require consuming more food than one

CHAPTER 1

Underweight: Definition

Underweight is a term used to describe a person whose body weight is lower than what is considered healthy for their age, height, and gender. It is often determined by calculating the Body Mass Index (BMI), which is a measure of body fat based on a person's height and weight.

A BMI below 18.5 is generally considered underweight. However, it is important to note that BMI is not always an accurate indicator of underweight, as it does not take into account factors such as muscle mass, bone density, and body composition.

Underweight can be caused by a variety of factors, including genetics, inadequate food intake, underlying medical conditions, and mental health disorders such as anorexia nervosa. It can also be the result of certain medications, such as chemotherapy drugs or those used to treat depression.

Being underweight can have negative effects on a person's health, including weakened immune system, increased risk of infections, and slower wound healing. It can also lead to malnutrition, which can cause a variety of health problems such as anemia, nutrient deficiencies, and stunted growth.

If a person is underweight, it is important to identify the underlying cause and work with a healthcare professional to develop a plan for reaching a healthy weight. This may include changes to the person's diet, increasing physical activity, and addressing any underlying medical or mental health conditions.

underweight is a term used to describe a person whose body weight is lower than what is considered healthy for their age, height, and gender. It can be caused by a variety of factors and can have negative effects on a person's health. Identifying the underlying cause and working with a healthcare professional is important for reaching a healthy weight and maintaining good health. understanding weight gain is essential for individuals who are underweight and seeking to gain weight in a healthy manner and individuals may face unique changes and challenges when trying to gain weight.

REASON WHY PEOPLE ARE UNDERWEIGHT

There are various reasons why some people are underweight, which can be classified into three main categories: medical, behavioral, and genetic factors.

Medical Factors

Certain medical conditions and illnesses can lead to being underweight, and such conditions are; hyperthyroidism, cancer, gastrointestinal disorders like celiac disease or Crohn's disease, and chronic infections such as tuberculosis or HIV. These conditions can cause a decreased appetite, malabsorption of nutrients, or an increased metabolic rate, which can result in weight loss.

Behavioral Factors

Poor dietary habits and inadequate caloric intake can also contribute to being underweight. Eating disorders such as anorexia nervosa or bulimia can lead to extreme weight loss due to an obsession with food and body image. Additionally, drug and alcohol abuse can lead to weight loss due to decreased appetite and malnourishment.

Genetic Factors

Genetics can also play a role in determining body weight. Some people may have a naturally high metabolism or a genetic predisposition towards being lean.

Additionally, socioeconomic factors can also influence a person's weight. Poverty and lack of access to nutritious food can lead to malnutrition and being underweight.

In order to address being underweight, it is important to identify the underlying cause. Medical conditions require proper diagnosis and treatment by a healthcare professional. Behavioral factors may require therapy and nutritional counseling to address the root cause of the issue. For genetic factors, individuals may benefit from working with a registered dietitian or physician to develop a healthy eating plan that is appropriate for their body type.

Being underweight can have negative health consequences and it is important to identify the underlying cause in order to address the issue and maintain a healthy weight.

Another problem that individuals face when trying to gain weight is social stigma. While being overweight is often stigmatized, being underweight can also be stigmatized. People may make comments or assumptions about a person's health or lifestyle based on their body size, which can be hurtful and discouraging. This can make it difficult for individuals to feel confident and motivated to gain weight.

Overall, being underweight can have negative health consequences and it is important to identify the underlying cause in order to address the issue and maintain a healthy weight.

CHAPTER 2

Natural Ways to Gain Weight

Some people may find it difficult to gain weight, particularly if they have a fast metabolism or a lack of appetite. While there are various supplements and weight gain products on the market, these options can be expensive and may have negative side effects. Fortunately, there are natural methods that can help individuals gain weight safely and effectively.

In the book "***Gain Body Weight & Confidence***" readers will learn about the different strategies that can be used to increase their body weight without relying on artificial supplements or processed foods. The book takes a holistic approach to weight gain, addressing factors such as nutrition, exercise, and sleep that can impact a person's ability to gain weight.

One of the main focuses of the book is on proper nutrition. The authors provide detailed information on the types of foods that are most beneficial for weight gain, as well as meal planning tips and recipes. They also discuss the importance of consuming enough protein, carbohydrates, and healthy fats to support muscle growth and overall health.

In addition to nutrition, the book also covers the role of exercise in weight gain. The authors provide guidance on strength training and other forms of exercise that can help individuals build muscle mass and improve their overall physical fitness. They also discuss the importance of rest and recovery for optimal results.

Overall, **_"Gain Body Weight & Confidence"_** is a comprehensive guide that can be a valuable resource for individuals who are looking to gain weight naturally and safely. Whether you're a hard gainer or simply looking to add some healthy weight to your frame, this book can provide the information and guidance you need to achieve your goals.

Setting realistic weight gain goals and tracking progress is important for individuals who are underweight and looking to improve their health. Here are some steps to help you set realistic weight gain goals and track your progress:

Determine your Target Weight

The first step is to determine your target weight, which should be realistic and achievable. You can use a body mass index (BMI) calculator to determine a healthy weight range based on your height and age.

Set a Realistic Timeline

Weight gain should be gradual and steady, typically 0.5-1 pound per week. Setting a realistic timeline can help you avoid frustration and disappointment.

Create a Meal Plan

You must consume more calories than you expend in order to acquire weight. A registered dietitian can help you create a meal plan that meets your calorie needs and includes nutrient-dense foods like lean protein, whole grains, fruits, and vegetables.

Exercise Regularly

Exercise can help build muscle mass and improve overall health. Resistance training and weightlifting can be particularly helpful for building muscle mass.

Track Your Progress

Keep track of your weight, calorie intake, and exercise routine in a journal or spreadsheet. This can help you identify trends and make adjustments to your plan as needed.

Make Adjustments as Needed

If you are not seeing progress, it may be necessary to make adjustments to your plan. You may need to increase your calorie intake or adjust your exercise routine to better support weight gain.

Stay Motivated

Weight gain can be challenging, and it's important to stay motivated and focused on your goals. Surround yourself with supportive friends and family members, and celebrate small milestones along the way.

Chapter 4

Nutrition for Underweight Individuals

Key considerations for nutrition in underweight individuals trying to gain weight.

For underweight people trying to gain weight, it is essential to consume a balanced diet that is rich in essential nutrients. The goal is to consume more calories than the body burns, in order to promote weight gain. Here are some key considerations for a nutrition plan for underweight individuals

Increase Calorie Intake

A calorie surplus is necessary for weight gain. The exact amount of calories needed will depend on the individual's body composition and activity level, but a general guideline is to consume 300-500 more calories than the body burns per day.

Eat Frequently

Eating small, frequent meals throughout the day can help increase calorie intake without feeling overly full.

Aim for 5-6 meals per day, with snacks in between.

Focus on nutrient-dense foods: Rather than relying on high-calorie junk food, it is important to choose nutrient-dense foods that provide the body with essential vitamins and minerals. Good options include whole grains, lean proteins, fruits, vegetables, and healthy fats.

Increase Protein Intake

Protein is essential for building and repairing muscle tissue, which is important for weight gain. Aim for 1-1.5 grams of protein per kilogram of body weight per day, with sources such as lean meat, fish, eggs, dairy, and plant-based proteins such as beans and tofu.

Choose Healthy Fats

Healthy fats are a good source of calories and essential fatty acids, which are important for overall health. Good options include nuts, seeds, avocado, olive oil, and fatty fish.

Stay Hydrated

Drinking plenty of water is important for overall health and can help prevent dehydration, which can negatively impact appetite and energy levels.

Understand, underweight individuals trying to gain weight should focus on consuming a balanced diet that is rich in calories, protein, nutrient-dense foods, healthy fats, and water. Consultation with a registered dietitian can also be helpful in developing an individualized nutrition plan.

Importance of Hydration And Meal Planning

Hydration and proper meal planning are crucial for underweight people for weight gain. Eating a diet that is rich in protein, complex carbohydrates, and healthy fats can help promote weight gain. Protein is essential for building and repairing muscle tissue, while carbohydrates provide the body with energy. Healthy fats are also necessary for proper bodily function and can help with weight gain. It is important to note that consuming too many unhealthy fats and simple carbohydrates can lead to weight gain in the form of fat, which is not ideal for those trying to gain weight.

Here are some of the key reasons you should hydrate and plan your meals:

Hydration Helps Maintain Bodily Functions

To keep your body functioning properly, stay moisturized. When you're dehydrated, your body can't function properly, and this can lead to fatigue, headaches, and other health problems. Drinking plenty of water helps keep your body hydrated and functioning at its best.

Proper Meal Planning Ensures Adequate Nutrient Intake

For underweight people, it's essential to consume enough calories and nutrients to gain weight and build muscle. Proper meal planning involves choosing nutrient-dense foods that are high in calories, protein, and healthy fats. This helps ensure that your body is getting the nutrients it needs to support weight gain and muscle growth.

Helps Maintain Energy Levels

When you're underweight, your body may not be getting enough energy from the food you eat, which can lead to fatigue and weakness. Proper meal planning and hydration can help maintain energy levels throughout the day, allowing you to be more active and productive.

Helps Improve Immune Function

Being underweight can weaken your immune system, making you more susceptible to illness and infection. Proper hydration and meal planning can help support immune function by providing the nutrients your body needs to stay healthy.

In summary, hydration and proper meal planning are essential for underweight people to maintain proper bodily functions, ensure adequate nutrient intake, maintain energy levels, and improve immune function. It's important to work with a healthcare professional or registered dietitian to develop a meal plan that meets your specific needs and goals.

BONUS

Breakfast at 8am Boosted My Performance

As a busy professional with a demanding schedule, I was always looking for ways to optimize my productivity and energy levels. I tried different diets, supplements, and workout routines, but nothing seemed to have a significant impact on my performance until I started eating exactly at 8 am every morning.

I had read about the benefits of intermittent fasting and how it could improve mental clarity, boost energy levels, and even lead to weight loss. However, I didn't want to skip meals or restrict my calorie intake, so I decided to try a different approach.

I started waking up at 6:30 am every day, which gave me plenty of time to prepare and enjoy a healthy breakfast before starting my day. I made sure to eat a balanced meal that included protein, healthy fats, and complex carbohydrates to keep me full and satisfied until lunchtime.

At first, it was challenging to stick to this routine, especially on weekends or when traveling. However, I noticed a significant difference in my energy levels and mental clarity within a week of starting this habit. I felt more focused, alert, and productive, and I could tackle my tasks with ease.

As time went by, I also noticed a positive impact on my physical health. I had more consistent energy levels throughout the day, which made it easier to stay active and exercise regularly. I also slept better at night, which improved my overall mood and wellbeing.

By the end of the first month, I had experienced a noticeable improvement in my productivity, creativity, and overall performance. I felt more confident in my abilities and was able to accomplish more in less time. I also felt happier and more fulfilled in both my personal and professional life.

Eating exactly at 8 am every morning has been a game-changer for me. It has helped me to optimize my physical and mental health, increase my productivity, and achieve my goals more efficiently. If you're looking for a simple yet effective way to improve your performance, I highly recommend trying this habit for yourself.

CHAPTER 5

Exercise for Underweight Individuals

For many people, gaining weight can be just as challenging as losing it. While there are numerous articles and advice available for people looking to lose weight, there is often less information for those looking to gain weight, especially for underweight individuals. While diet plays a significant role in weight gain, exercise can be a valuable tool in achieving weight gain goals, particularly for underweight individuals. In this article, we will discuss how exercise can help improve weight gain goals for underweight people.

First and foremost, it is important to understand that weight gain is primarily dependent on calorie intake. To gain weight, you need to consume more calories than you burn. However, simply consuming more calories is not enough. You need to ensure that the calories you consume are healthy and nutritious, providing your body with the necessary nutrients to build muscle and gain weight. This is where exercise comes in.

Strength Training

Strength training is one of the most effective ways to build muscle and gain weight. Lifting weights or using resistance machines causes tiny tears in the muscle fibers, which the body then repairs and strengthens, resulting in increased muscle mass. This increased muscle mass contributes to weight gain and also boosts metabolism, allowing you to burn more calories throughout the day.

Resistance Training

Resistance training can also help underweight individuals gain weight by increasing their appetite. Exercise increases the production of hormones, such as testosterone and growth hormone, which can stimulate appetite. By stimulating the appetite, resistance training can help underweight individuals consume the extra calories they need to gain weight.

Cardiovascular Exercise

Cardiovascular exercise, such as running, cycling, or swimming, can also be beneficial for weight gain. While cardio burns calories and may seem counterintuitive to weight gain goals, it can improve overall fitness, endurance, and energy levels, allowing you to exercise for longer and more intensely during strength and resistance training, ultimately leading to greater muscle gains and weight gain.

Consistency

Finally, it is essential to be consistent with exercise. Regular exercise can help build muscle and increase appetite, but it needs to be done consistently to see results. Start with a manageable workout routine and gradually increase the intensity and duration over time. As with any exercise program, it is essential to listen to your body and adjust your routine accordingly.

In conclusion, exercise can be a valuable tool for underweight individuals looking to gain weight. Strength and resistance training can help build muscle and increase appetite, while cardiovascular exercise can improve overall fitness and endurance, ultimately leading to greater muscle gains and weight gain. However, exercise alone is not enough to achieve weight gain goals. A healthy and nutritious diet, providing the body with the necessary nutrients, is also crucial. With a combination of exercise and a healthy diet, underweight individuals can achieve their weight gain goals and improve their overall health and wellbeing.

Chapter6

Underweight Lifestyle Changes

Being underweight can be just as unhealthy as being overweight. People who are underweight may have a weakened immune system, decreased muscle mass, and may be at a higher risk of malnutrition and chronic diseases. Therefore, gaining weight in a healthy and sustainable way can help underweight individuals improve their overall health and wellbeing. However, simply increasing calorie intake without making other lifestyle changes may not be enough to achieve this goal.

To gain weight, underweight people need to create a calorie surplus by consuming more calories than they burn. However, it's important to do this in a healthy way by focusing on nutrient-dense foods such as lean proteins, whole grains, fruits, and vegetables. Eating a balanced and varied diet will help ensure that the body is getting all the nutrients it needs to function properly and support weight gain. Additionally, incorporating resistance training and weightlifting into a regular exercise routine can help build muscle mass and increase overall weight.

In addition to dietary changes and exercise, it's also important for underweight individuals to make other lifestyle changes to support weight gain. These changes may include getting adequate sleep, managing stress levels, and reducing alcohol and tobacco consumption. Sleep plays a vital role in the body's ability to repair and recover, and inadequate sleep can disrupt hormonal balance and negatively impact weight gain efforts. Stress can also interfere with weight gain by increasing the body's production of cortisol, a hormone that can lead to muscle breakdown and decreased appetite. Finally, excessive alcohol and tobacco consumption can negatively impact appetite and interfere with nutrient absorption, making it harder to gain weight in a healthy way.

In conclusion, underweight individuals looking to gain weight need to make a variety of lifestyle changes in addition to increasing their calorie intake. A balanced and nutrient-dense diet, regular exercise, adequate sleep, stress management, and reducing alcohol and tobacco consumption are all important factors in supporting healthy weight gain. By making these lifestyle changes, underweight individuals can not only gain weight but also improve their overall health and wellbeing.

Supplement for Underweight People

The idea of underweight people taking supplements for weight gain is a common one. Many people who are underweight, whether due to illness, genetics, or poor eating habits, may struggle to gain weight despite their best efforts. In these cases, supplements can be a useful tool for increasing calorie intake and promoting weight gain. However, as with any supplement or dietary intervention, there are both potential benefits and drawbacks to consider.

One potential benefit of using supplements for weight gain is that they can provide a quick and convenient source of extra calories. Many weight gain supplements are designed to be high in calories and protein, which can help individuals meet their daily calorie and nutrient needs without having to consume large quantities of food. This can be particularly helpful for people who struggle with poor appetite or who have difficulty eating enough to gain weight.

In addition, some weight gain supplements may contain specific nutrients that can be beneficial for promoting weight gain. For example, some supplements contain Creatine, which has been shown to increase muscle mass and strength in some individuals. Others may contain omega-3 fatty acids, which can help support healthy weight gain and promote overall health.

However, it is important to note that taking supplements for weight gain is not without risks. For one, many weight gain supplements are high in sugar and may contribute to unhealthy weight gain if consumed in excess. In addition, some supplements may contain ingredients that can be harmful if taken in large quantities or in combination with certain medications.

Furthermore, relying too heavily on supplements for weight gain can lead to an unbalanced diet and may prevent individuals from getting the nutrients they need from whole foods. While supplements can be a useful tool for promoting weight gain, they should not be relied upon as a substitute for a healthy, balanced diet.

Overall, the decision to take supplements for weight gain should be made in consultation with a healthcare professional or registered dietitian. These professionals can help individuals determine whether supplements are a good choice for their particular needs and can provide guidance on safe and effective supplement use.

That being said, it is important to note that healthy, whole foods should always be the first choice for promoting weight gain and overall health. Eating a balanced diet that includes plenty of nutrient-dense foods like fruits, vegetables, lean proteins, and whole grains can help individuals meet their calorie and nutrient needs in a way that promotes overall health and well-being.

In addition, eating whole foods can help individuals develop healthy eating habits and can reduce the risk of nutrient deficiencies and other health problems.

The idea of underweight people taking supplements for weight gain is a common one, but it is important to weigh the potential benefits and drawbacks before making a decision. While supplements can be a useful tool for promoting weight gain, they should not be relied upon as a substitute for a healthy, balanced diet. Consulting with a healthcare professional or registered dietitian can help individuals determine whether supplements are a good choice for their particular needs, and can provide guidance on safe and effective supplement use. Ultimately, healthy, whole foods should always be the first choice for promoting weight gain and overall health.

Chapter 7

Challenges of Gaining Weight

Gaining weight can be just as challenging as losing weight, and while the focus of weight management may be on losing weight, it's important to acknowledge the struggles that come with gaining weight. There are several challenges that people may face when trying to gain weight, which we will discuss below.

A Fast Metabolism

One of the most significant challenges people face when trying to gain weight is having a fast metabolism. A fast metabolism means that your body burns calories quickly, making it harder to gain weight. Even if you eat more calories than your body needs, your fast metabolism can quickly burn off the excess calories, making it challenging to gain weight.

Lack of Appetite

Another challenge people may face is a lack of appetite. Some people simply do not feel hungry or have a smaller appetite, making it hard to consume the necessary calories to gain weight. Moreover, if someone feels full quickly, they may struggle to eat enough calories throughout the day to gain weight.

Busy Schedule

People with a busy schedule may find it hard to gain weight. The hustle and bustle of everyday life can leave little time for cooking and meal planning. This can make it challenging to consume the right amount of calories and nutrients needed to gain weight.

Medical Conditions

Certain medical conditions can also make it challenging to gain weight. For example, people with hyperthyroidism may have a fast metabolism, making it harder to gain weight. Moreover, medical conditions that affect the digestive system, such as Crohn's disease, may also impact nutrient absorption, making it harder to gain weight.

Lack of Knowledge

Gaining weight requires a lot of knowledge and planning. People who lack knowledge about nutrition and calorie intake may find it challenging to consume the right foods and the right amount of calories. Without proper knowledge, they may consume too many calories from unhealthy sources, leading to negative health outcomes.

Fear of Unhealthy Eating

People who want to gain weight may fear eating unhealthy foods or eating too much. They may worry that consuming too much food or consuming unhealthy foods will negatively impact their health. This fear may prevent them from consuming enough calories and nutrients to gain weight.

Financial Constraints

Eating healthy and gaining weight can be expensive. People who are on a tight budget may find it challenging to purchase healthy, high-calorie foods. This can limit their food options and make it harder to consume enough calories and nutrients to gain weight.

Gaining weight is just as challenging as losing weight, and there are several challenges people may face when trying to gain weight. A fast metabolism, a lack of appetite, a busy schedule, medical conditions, lack of knowledge, fear of unhealthy eating, and financial constraints are some of the most common challenges people may encounter. However, with proper knowledge and planning, people can overcome these challenges and gain weight in a healthy way.

Chapter 8

Positive Mindset and Self-Care

Maintaining a healthy weight is an important aspect of leading a healthy lifestyle, but it can be a challenging task for many people. For those who struggle with weight gain, it's essential to adopt a positive mindset and engage in self-care practices to promote long-term success. In this article, we'll explore why a positive mindset and self-care are crucial for achieving and maintaining a healthy weight.

Importance of Positive Mindset

A positive mindset is critical when it comes to weight gain because it can help individuals stay motivated, manage stress, and overcome obstacles. When individuals approach weight gain with a negative mindset, they may feel defeated before they even begin. Negative self-talk and limiting beliefs can be a significant barrier to weight loss success. However, adopting a positive mindset can help individuals reframe their thoughts and beliefs and approach weight gain with a can-do attitude.

Here are a few ways a positive mindset can help individuals achieve and maintain a healthy weight

Stay Motivated

Motivation is a crucial factor when it comes to weight gain. It can be challenging to stay motivated when progress is slow or when individuals face setbacks. However, a positive mindset can help individuals stay motivated by focusing on their progress and accomplishments rather than their setbacks. By celebrating small wins and focusing on the positive, individuals can stay motivated and on track towards their weight gain goals.

Manage Stress

Stress can be a significant factor in weight gain. When individuals experience stress, they may turn to food for comfort or engage in other unhealthy habits that can lead to weight gain. However, a positive mindset can help individuals manage stress by adopting healthy coping mechanisms such as exercise, mindfulness, and meditation.

Overcome Obstacles

Obstacles are a natural part of the weight gain journey. However, a positive mindset can help individuals overcome obstacles by reframing challenges as opportunities for growth. Rather than getting discouraged by setbacks or challenges, individuals with a positive mindset can use these experiences as an opportunity to learn, grow, and improve.

Importance of Self-Care

Self-care is another critical aspect of weight gain. When individuals prioritize self-care, they are more likely to make healthy choices and take care of their bodies. Self-care practices can help individuals reduce stress, improve sleep, and promote overall well-being.

Here are a few ways self-care can help individuals achieve and maintain a healthy weight

Reduce Stress

Stress is a significant factor in weight gain. When individuals experience chronic stress, it can lead to increased cortisol levels, which can contribute to weight gain. However, self-care practices such as meditation, exercise, and spending time in nature can help reduce stress and promote overall well-being.

Improve Sleep

Sleep is another critical factor in weight gain. When individuals don't get enough sleep, it can lead to increased hunger, decreased metabolism, and impaired decision-making. However, self-care practices such as establishing a consistent sleep routine, avoiding screens before bedtime, and creating a comfortable sleep environment can promote better sleep and support weight gain goals.

Promote Overall Well-Being

Self-care practices can also promote overall well-being, which is essential for achieving and maintaining a healthy weight. When individuals prioritize self-care, they are more likely to make healthy choices, engage in physical activity, and take care of their bodies. Self-care can also help individuals reduce stress, improve sleep, and promote positive mental health, all of which are crucial for weight gain success.

Achieving and maintaining a healthy weight can be a challenging task, but a positive mindset and self-care practices can make all the difference. By adopting a can-do attitude, reframing negative thoughts, and focusing on the positive, individuals can stay motivated and overcome obstacles on their weight gain journey. Similarly, by prioritizing self-care practices such as exercise, mindfulness, and sleep,

CHAPTER 9

Healthy Foods for Weight Gain

While many people struggle to lose weight, there are others who are looking to gain weight in a healthy way. Adding certain foods to your diet can help you reach your weight gain goals without sacrificing your overall health. Here are ten natural, healthy foods that can help you put on some extra pounds.

Avocado

Avocado is a great source of healthy fats, which can help increase your calorie intake without filling you up. In fact, a single avocado contains about 320 calories, making it one of the most calorie-dense fruits out there. Avocados are also rich in fiber, potassium, and vitamins C, K, and B6.

Nuts

Nuts are an excellent source of healthy fats, protein, and fiber. They are also calorie-dense, making them a great choice for those looking to gain weight. Almonds, cashews, and peanuts are all great options. Just be sure to choose unsalted nuts to avoid consuming too much sodium.

Whole Grains

Whole grains are an excellent source of complex carbohydrates, which provide sustained energy throughout the day. They are also rich in fiber, vitamins, and minerals. Some good options include brown rice, quinoa, and whole grain bread.

Cheese

Cheese is a great source of protein and calcium, and it's also calorie-dense. Just be mindful of your portion sizes, as cheese can be high in saturated fat. Opt for low-fat or reduced-fat versions whenever possible.

Peanut Butter

Peanut butter is a great source of healthy fats, protein, and fiber. It's also calorie-dense, making it a great choice for those looking to gain weight. Just be sure to choose natural peanut butter without added sugars or oils.

Dried Fruit

Dried fruit is a great way to add some extra calories to your diet. It's also a good source of fiber, vitamins, and minerals. Just be sure to choose unsweetened dried fruit to avoid consuming too much added sugar.

Milk

Milk is an excellent source of calcium, protein, and vitamin D. It's also calorie-dense, making it a great choice for those looking to gain weight. Choose low-fat or skim milk to avoid consuming too much saturated fat.

Olive Oil

Olive oil is a great source of healthy fats, which can help increase your calorie intake without filling you up. It's also rich in antioxidants and anti-inflammatory compounds, which can help reduce the risk of chronic diseases.

Eggs

Eggs are an excellent source of protein, healthy fats, and vitamins and minerals. They are also calorie-dense, making them a great choice for those looking to gain weight. Just be mindful of your portion sizes, as eggs can be high in cholesterol.

Lean Meats

Lean meats, such as chicken, turkey, and lean beef, are a great source of protein and essential nutrients like iron and zinc. They are also calorie-dense, making them a great choice for those looking to gain weight. Just be sure to choose lean cuts of meat to avoid consuming too much saturated fat.

Gaining weight in a healthy way involves adding nutrient-dense, calorie-dense foods to your diet. The ten foods listed above are all great choices for those looking to gain weight while still maintaining a healthy diet. Remember to eat a variety of foods and to consult with a healthcare professional before making any significant changes to your diet.

So if you are looking for a way to take your health and weight gain to the next level, then this is the part you have been waiting for. Get ready to discover the natural game changer foods that will revolutionize the way you eat and live.

Whole grains (oats, quinoa, brown rice)

Lean protein sources (chicken breast, fish, turkey, tofu)

Dairy products (milk, cheese, yogurt)

Fruits (bananas, berries, dried fruit)

Vegetables (sweet potatoes, broccoli, spinach)

However, if you're looking for some game changer foods for weight gain, here are a few options;

Greek Yogurt

Greek yogurt is a great source of protein and can be used as a base for smoothies or mixed with nuts and fruit for a high-calorie snack.

Hummus

Hummus is made from chickpeas, which are a great source of fiber and protein. You can dip vegetables or crackers in it for a healthy snack.

Quinoa

Quinoa is a whole grain that's high in protein and fiber. It can be used as a base for salads or mixed with vegetables and a protein source for a hearty meal.

Salmon

Salmon is a great source of omega-3 fatty acids and protein, and can be baked, grilled or broiled for a healthy and satisfying meal.

Sweet Potatoes

Sweet potatoes are a great source of fiber

CHAPTER 10

Weight Gain Secret Changer

Cornmeal Porridge

cornmeal porridge or maize meal, is a popular staple food. It is made by grinding dried corn kernels into a fine powder, which is then mixed with water and cooked over low heat until it forms a thick, smooth porridge.

Pap can be a helpful food for those looking to gain weight because it is high in calories, carbohydrates, and nutrients. One cup of cooked pap contains around 150-200 calories, which makes it a good addition to a high-calorie diet. It also contains a significant amount of carbohydrates, which are an important energy source for the body.

In addition to being calorie-dense and high in carbs, pap is also a good source of vitamins and minerals, including iron, magnesium, and vitamin B6. These nutrients are important for maintaining good health and supporting the body's metabolic processes.

Preparation

you will need:

1 cup of maize meal

2 cups of water

A pinch of salt (optional)

Instructions

- Bring the water to a boil in a medium-sized saucepan.

- In a separate bowl, mix the maize meal with a little bit of water to make a smooth paste.

- Slowly pour the maize meal mixture into the boiling water, stirring constantly to prevent lumps from forming.

- Reduce the heat to low and continue to stir the pap until it thickens and pulls away from the sides of the pot.

- Cover the pot and let the pap simmer for an additional 5-10 minutes.

- Remove from heat and let it cool for a few minutes before serving.

You can serve pap as a side dish with a protein source such as grilled chicken, fish, or beans to make a complete meal. You can also add milk, butter, honey, or sugar to the pap to make it more flavorful and increase its calorie content.

Cereal pudding

This is made from maize or corn. It is a type of porridge that is often consumed as a breakfast food or a snack. Fermentation is a process where microorganisms break down the carbohydrates in the maize, making it easier to digest and increasing its nutrient availability. Here are some ways fermented pap can help in adding weight:

Fermented Maize Is High in Calories
Fermentation increases the calorie content of the maize, making it a high-

calorie food. This makes it an excellent food for those looking to gain weight.

It Is Rich in Nutrients

Fermentation breaks down the complex carbohydrates in maize into simpler forms, making it easier to digest and increasing its nutrient availability. Fermented pap is rich in vitamins and minerals, including vitamin B, iron, and calcium.

It Aids Digestion

The fermentation process breaks down the complex carbohydrates in maize, making it easier to digest. This can help improve digestive health, which is important for overall weight gain.

The process of preparing fermented pap is quite simple. Here's how it's done;

Preparation

- Soak the maize in water for about 2-3 days to allow it to soften.

- Drain the water and grind the maize into a fine paste.

- Add water to the paste and stir until it forms a smooth consistency.

- Place the mixture in a container and cover it with a clean cloth.

- Leave it to ferment for about 1-2 days, depending on the desired level of fermentation.

- Once fermented, stir the mixture to break up any lumps and boil it for about 10-15 minutes.

- Allow it to cool and serve with milk, sugar or any other preferred toppings.

In summary, fermented Maize or Corn is a high-calorie, nutrient-rich food that can aid in weight gain. Its preparation is simple and involves soaking, grinding, fermenting, and boiling maize to create a delicious and healthy porridge.

Yam Tubers for Weight Gain

Yams are a nutritious root vegetable that can be beneficial for underweight people who are looking to gain weight in a healthy way. Here are some ways that yams can help;

High in Carbohydrates

Yams are a good source of carbohydrates, which are essential for energy and can help in gaining weight. They are also high in dietary fiber, which can aid in digestion and improve bowel movements.

Rich in Vitamins and Minerals

Yams are packed with vitamins and minerals, including vitamin C, potassium, and manganese, which can help improve overall health and well-being.

Anti-Inflammatory Properties

Yams contain compounds that have anti-inflammatory properties, which can help reduce inflammation in the body and support a healthy immune system.

To prepare yam tubers for weight gain, there are a variety of recipes you can try. Here's one simple recipe;

Ingredients

2 medium-sized yams

2 tablespoons of olive oil

Salt and pepper to taste

Herbs and spices of your choice (optional)

Instructions

- Pre-heat your oven to 400°F (200°C).

- Wash and peel the yams, then cut them into small pieces.

- In a bowl, toss the yams with olive oil, salt, pepper, and any other herbs or spices you prefer.

- Spread the yam pieces in a single layer on a baking sheet.

- Bake the yams for about 25-30 minutes, or until they are tender and lightly browned.

- Serve the roasted yams as a side dish, or add them to salads, stews, or soups for extra nutrition and flavor.

Other ways to enjoy yams include boiling, frying, or mashing them. You can also use yam flour to make pancakes, bread, or other baked goods. Just be sure to balance your yam intake with other healthy foods, such as lean proteins, fruits, and vegetables, to ensure a balanced diet.

Tom brown pudding

Tom brown is a thick brown nutritious and healthy meal that can help in adding weight for underweight people. Tom brown is made from roasted grains such as maize, millet, and sorghum. Millet is a good source of protein, fiber, vitamins, and minerals, making it a great food for those looking to gain weight.

The fermentation process increases the nutritional value of the millet, making it easier to digest and absorb nutrients. Fermentation also increases the availability of micronutrients such as iron and zinc. These micronutrients are essential for proper growth and development and can help underweight individuals gain weight.

To prepare fermented tom brown made with millet, follow these steps;

Ingredients

2 cups of millet

1 tablespoon of yoghurt or buttermilk (as a starter culture)

Water

Instructions

- Rinse the millet in water and then soak it in water for about 8-12 hours.

- Drain the water and spread the millet on a clean cloth or tray to dry.

- Roast the millet on low heat until it turns golden brown. Make sure to stir continuously to prevent burning.

- Grind the roasted millet into a fine powder.

- Add water to the powdered millet to form a thick paste.

- In a clean bowl, mix the millet paste with the yoghurt or buttermilk starter culture.

- Cover the bowl with a clean cloth and leave it to ferment for 24-48 hours in a warm place. The longer the fermentation process, the more sour the taste.

- After fermentation, stir the mixture and sieve out the chaff.

Store the fermented tom brown in an airtight container in a cool, dry place.

To prepare fermented tom brown for consumption, mix the fermented tom brown with hot water or milk until it forms a smooth porridge. You can sweeten it with honey or sugar to taste.

Overall, fermented tom brown made with millet is a great food for adding weight in underweight individuals. It is a nutrient-dense food that can provide the necessary nutrients for proper growth and development.

Sweet Potato Weight Gain

Sweet potatoes can be a healthy and nutritious addition to an underweight person's diet to help them gain weight. Sweet potatoes are high in carbohydrates, which are essential for energy and weight gain. They are also rich in fiber, vitamins, and minerals, which are important for overall health.

Here are some ways to prepare sweet potatoes;

Baked Sweet Potatoes

Preheat the oven to 400°F. Wash and dry sweet potatoes, pierce them with a fork, and place them on a baking sheet. Bake for 45-60 minutes or until tender. Enjoy as a side dish or snack.

Sweet Potato Fries

Cut sweet potatoes into thin strips, toss them with a little bit of olive oil, salt, and pepper, and bake them in the oven at 425°F for 15-20 minutes, flipping once halfway through. Enjoy as a snack or side dish.

Mashed Sweet Potatoes

Boil sweet potatoes until tender, then mash them with a fork or potato masher. Add a little bit of butter, salt, and pepper for flavor. Enjoy as a side dish.

Sweet Potato Smoothie

Blend cooked sweet potatoes with milk, vanilla extract, and a sweetener of your choice (such as honey or maple syrup). Enjoy as a breakfast or snack.

It's important to note that while sweet potatoes can help with weight gain, it's important to consume them as part of a balanced diet that includes protein and healthy fats. Consult with a healthcare professional or registered dietitian to determine the appropriate diet and caloric intake for your specific needs.

Gruel (Made with Millet or Sorghum)

Gruel beverage is made from grains like millet, sorghum, and corn. It is a rich source of nutrients and can be helpful in adding weight for underweight people. Here's how;

High Calorie Content

Gruel is a high-calorie drink that can help underweight people to increase their calorie intake. It contains up to 400 calories per serving, which is essential for weight gain.

Rich in Nutrients

Gruel is rich in nutrients like protein, carbohydrates, and fiber, which are essential for weight gain. It also contains vitamins and minerals like iron, calcium, and magnesium.

Promotes digestion

Gruel is fermented, which makes it rich in probiotics that aid digestion. Good digestion is essential for nutrient absorption, and with better absorption, underweight people can gain weight faster.

To prepare this kind of Gruel, you will need the following ingredients;

2 cups of millet or sorghum

1/4 cup of peanuts

1/4 cup of ginger

1/2 cup of sugar

1/2 teaspoon of salt

5 cups of water

Directions

- Rinse the millet and soak it in water for about 24 hours. Drain the water and let the millet dry.

- Roast the peanuts and ginger in a pan until they are brown. Remove them from the heat and set aside.

- Grind the millet, peanuts, and ginger in a blender or food processor until they become a smooth powder.

- Add water to the powder and mix well. Leave the mixture to ferment for about 24 to 48 hours.

- After fermentation, strain the mixture to remove any lumps or residue.

- Add sugar and salt to the mixture and mix well.

- Serve the gruel chilled or with ice.

Note, You can adjust the quantity of sugar and salt to your taste preference.

In summary, gruel can be a helpful addition to the diet of underweight people looking to add weight. Its high-calorie content and rich nutrient profile make it a good option for weight gain. To prepare this type of gruel, you need millet, peanuts, ginger, sugar, salt, and water.

Nut Butter

Nut butter can be a valuable addition to the diet of underweight people looking to gain weight because it is high in calories and healthy fats. Nut butter is made by grinding nuts into a smooth paste, which can be spread on bread, crackers, or used as a dip for fruits and vegetables.

To make nut butter, you will need a food processor or blender and a selection of nuts, such as almonds, cashews, peanuts, or hazelnuts. Begin by roasting the nuts in the oven at 350°F for 10-15 minutes or until they become fragrant and slightly browned. Next, place the nuts into the food processor or blender and pulse until they become a smooth paste. You can add a pinch of salt or a drizzle of honey to enhance the flavor if desired.

To serve nut butter with 2 rolls of bread, begin by selecting your favorite bread rolls and cutting them in half. Spread a generous amount of nut butter on each half, and enjoy as is or add your favorite toppings such as sliced banana, honey, or jam.

It's essential to remember that while nut butter can be an excellent way to add calories and healthy fats to your diet, it should be consumed in moderation as it is high in calories. Pairing nut butter with whole-grain bread rolls can provide additional fiber and nutrients that can support healthy weight gain. Additionally, it's essential to maintain a balanced diet and incorporate a variety of nutrient-dense foods to support optimal health.

Beans and ripe plantain

Cooked beans and ripe plantains are both nutritious foods that can help underweight people gain weight in a healthy way. Here are some ways that these foods can help;

High in Calories

Both cooked beans and ripe plantains are high in calories, which can help underweight people consume more energy than they are burning. A cup of cooked beans contains about 220 calories, while a medium-sized ripe plantain contains about 200 calories.

Good Source of Protein

Beans are an excellent source of plant-based protein, with a cup of cooked beans containing around 15 grams of protein. Plantains also contain a small amount of protein. Consuming adequate protein is important for building and repairing muscles, which can help underweight individuals gain healthy weight.

High in Fiber

Both cooked beans and ripe plantains are high in fiber, which can aid digestion and promote satiety. This can help underweight individuals consume more food and feel full for longer periods of time.

Rich in Vitamins and Minerals

Beans and plantains are both rich in vitamins and minerals that are essential for overall health. For example, beans are a good source of iron, folate, and potassium, while plantains are a good source of vitamin C and vitamin A.

To incorporate cooked beans and ripe plantains into your diet, consider adding them to meals like rice dishes, stews, or salads. You could also eat them as a snack or side dish. Be sure to also consume a balanced diet that includes other nutrient-dense foods like fruits, vegetables, and lean protein sources to support your overall health and weight gain goals.

Bonus

Banana, coconut oil, peanut butter, Greek yogurt (Mixed Together)

Consume once or twice a day, it is highly fatty.

Bananas, coconut oil, peanut butter, and Greek yogurt are all excellent foods that can help underweight individuals to gain weight in a healthy way. These ingredients are all high in calories, healthy fats, and protein, which are essential for weight gain. Here's how you can mix or blend them together to create a tasty and nutritious snack;

Ingredients

1 ripe banana

1 tablespoon of coconut oil

1 tablespoon of peanut butter

1/2 cup of Greek yogurt

Instructions

- Peel the banana and cut it into small pieces.

- Add the banana, coconut oil, peanut butter, and Greek yogurt to a blender or food processor.

- Blend the ingredients until smooth and creamy.

- If the mixture is too thick, add a little bit of milk or water to thin it out.

- To serve with 2 rolls of bread and a boiled egg, follow these instructions:

Ingredients

2 rolls of bread

1 boiled egg

Banana, coconut oil, peanut butter, and Greek yogurt mixture

Instructions

- Cut the rolls of bread in half and toast them.

- Spread the banana, coconut oil, peanut butter, and Greek yogurt mixture on each half of the rolls.

- Peel the boiled egg and slice it into rounds.

- Place the egg slices on top of the mixture.

- Serve immediately and enjoy!

This snack provides a good balance of carbohydrates, healthy fats, and protein, making it an ideal option for underweight individuals who are looking to gain weight. The rolls of bread provide carbs, while the boiled egg adds protein. The mixture of banana, coconut oil, peanut butter, and

Greek yogurt is high in healthy fats and protein, which are essential for weight gain.

You can also increase the quantity of the ingredients if you wish to store in freezer and take a glass everyday.

Conclusion

In conclusion, weight gain is a complex topic that affects many people, and this book has delved into the reasons why some individuals struggle with being underweight. We have explored the importance of proper nutrition and exercise for gaining weight in a healthy manner, as well as the challenges that come with trying to gain weight.

One of the main reasons some people are underweight is due to a high metabolism, which makes it difficult to gain weight even when consuming a surplus of calories. In addition, genetics can play a role in determining an individual's body type and ability to gain weight. However, it is important to note that being underweight can also be a symptom of underlying medical conditions, and it is important to consult a healthcare professional if one is experiencing unexplained weight loss.

Nutrition is a crucial aspect of weight gain, and this book has emphasized the importance of consuming a diet that is high in calories and protein. Eating frequent meals and snacks throughout the day can help increase calorie intake, and incorporating healthy fats such as nuts and avocado can help boost overall calorie intake as well. It is important to note, however, that gaining weight in a healthy manner involves consuming nutrient-dense foods rather than relying solely on high-calorie junk food.

Exercise can also play a role in weight gain by building muscle mass, which contributes to overall weight gain. Resistance training such as weight lifting and bodyweight exercises can help increase muscle mass and promote weight gain. However, it is important to approach exercise in a balanced manner and not over-exercise, as this can lead to burnout and injury.

The challenges of gaining weight are not to be underestimated, as it can be a difficult and frustrating process. Some individuals may struggle with appetite and find it difficult to consume enough calories, while others may face societal pressures to maintain a certain body type. Additionally, gaining weight can be a slow process, and it is important to remain patient and consistent in order to see results.

Gaining weight in a healthy and sustainable manner involves a combination of proper nutrition and exercise, as well as patience and persistence. While the challenges of weight gain may seem daunting, it is important to prioritize one's health and well-being over societal pressures or unrealistic expectations. By following the advice and tips outlined in this book, individuals struggling with being underweight can take steps towards achieving their weight gain goals in a safe and healthy manner.

9 798389 977143